Paleo Diet Smoothies for Strength

Smoothie Recipes and Nutrition Plan for Strength Athletes & Bodybuilders - Achieve Peak Health, Performance and Physique (Food for Fitness Series)

Lars Andersen

Published by Nordic Standard Publishing

Atlanta, Georgia USA

ISBN 978-1-484145-26-5

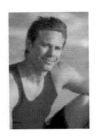

Lars Andersen

Copyright © 2012 Lars Andersen

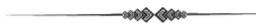

What Our Readers Are Saying

"These are such a clever and convenient way to get meet my protein needs"

★★★★☆ **Kai E. Young (Boise, ID)**

"Lot's of good information and tasty recipes. Highly recommended"

★★★★☆ **Brian L. Hill (Willoughby, OH)**

"All natural and they work out cheaper than the store-bought protein powders - awesome!"

★★★★☆ **Peter M. Cesar (Chicago, IL)**

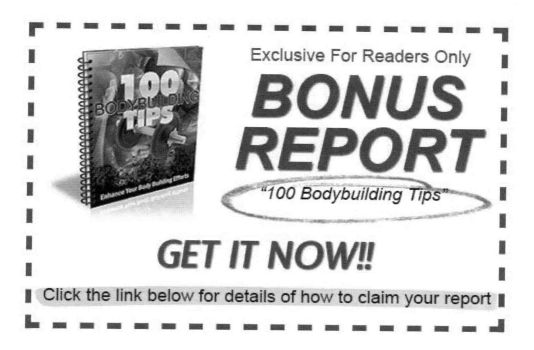

Exclusive Bonus Download: 100 Bodybuilding Tips

People all over the world, not just men, are interested in bulking up through bodybuilding exercises. This area used to be the exclusive domain of men, but now women are becoming serious bodybuilders, whether competing in body sculpting competitions or getting more muscles to lift more weight. Whatever the reason, bodybuilding is one of the hot topics being researched online today.

But just like any exercise or diet routine, bodybuilding requires discipline. You need to take stock of yourself first to see if you have the commitment that it's going to take. " 100 Bodybuilding Tips " will show you how to attain the right mindset, how to prepare yourself physically, ways to burn fat and build cardio strength, and pitfalls to avoid in establishing a bodybuilding routine. These tips contain the information that you'll need to get started on a serious regimen, all the while avoiding injury and developing muscle mass safely in harmony with your body's processes. You'll get information about which exercises produce which results, and how to avoid the common myths that many people believe about gaining muscle through bodybuilding.

People begin to lose muscle mass as they approach middle age. Many people who enjoyed the benefits of strength in their youth find themselves with backaches and other ailments which could be alleviated with stronger, healthier muscles. Whether you want to be on the cover of a fitness magazine or just enjoy a higher quality of life, get " 100 Bodybuilding Tips " and learn how to make a change in your life today.

Go to the end of this book for the download link for this Bonus!

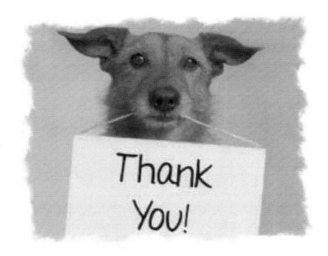

Thank you for downloading my book. Please REVIEW this book on Amazon. I need your feedback to make the next edition better. Thank you so much!

Books by Lars Andersen

The Smoothies for Runners Book

Juices for Runners

Smoothies for Cyclists

Juices for Cyclists

Palio Diet for Cyclists

Smoothies for Triathletes

Juices for Triathletes

Palio Diet for Triathletes

Smoothies for Strength

Juices for Strength

Palio Diet for Strength

Palio Diet Smoothies for Strength

Smoothies for Golfers

Juices for Golfers

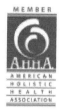

Table of Contents

Disclaimer

Paleo Diet Smoothies for Strength Training and Muscle Building

"Life expectancy would grow by leaps and bounds if green vegetables smelled as good as bacon" – Doug Larson

The current US Department of Agriculture (USDA) healthy eating guidelines promote a balanced daily diet consisting of 60 percent carbohydrates, 30 percent fats, and 10 percent protein. Switching from USDA recommendations to a Paleo diet will generally lead to an increase in your overall protein and fat intake and a drop in your overall carbohydrate intake. However, your main sources of carbohydrates will be fruits and vegetables, meaning that you will gain a plentiful supply of healthful micro-nutrients, and your main sources of protein and fats will be lean meats with low levels of saturated fat, and fish with high levels of omega-3 essential fatty acids.

The Paleo diet can be summed up in one simple rule of thumb proposed by Paleo advocates; "If it's in a box, you shouldn't be eating it." Paleo is the common name given to the Paleolithic diet, so named because of its similarities to the diet of our hunter-gatherer ancestors some 2.5 million years ago in the Paleolithic Era. In essence, it's a diet that revolves around eating foods which occur naturally and avoiding foods which would be unrecognizable to a Paleolithic caveman! Cutting all "modern" foodstuffs from your diet, including all forms of grain as well as highly processed convenience foods, leaves a diet of all natural foodstuffs, for example:

- **Meat** – grass-fed rather than grain-fed animal sources.
- **Fowl** – chicken, turkey, duck, and game birds.
- **Fish** – wild fish rather than farmed fish as the latter can contain unhealthy levels of mercury and other toxins.
- **Eggs** – organic, free range and ideally omega-3 enriched.
- **Vegetables** – excluding modern farmed varieties.
- **Oils** – any natural source such as coconut oil, walnut oil, or avocado oil.
- **Fruits** – berries in particular and other fruits in moderation.
- **Nuts** – excluding peanuts.
- **Tubers** – sweet potatoes and yams in particular.

There is no *one* Paleo diet, and it's important to note that a Paleo-based diet is not necessarily a "low-carb diet" as such. Some hunter-gatherer populations would have survived and thrived on a low-carb diet; others would have lived equally well on a high-carb diet of fish, tubers, and coconut. An important element of all Paleo-based diets is that locally sourced organic produce should make up the bulk of your daily food intake whenever possible. However, this can prove expensive in some areas of today's world, so aiming to eat the best quality produce you can afford is an important step in terms of getting the most from a Paleo diet.

Paleo Fuel Sources

Paleo "purists" eat only foods which can be hunted, fished or gathered. Foods include meat, offal, seafood, eggs, insects, fruits, nuts, seeds, vegetables, mushrooms, herbs and spices. Excluded foods include grains, legumes – beans and peanuts – dairy products, refined sugar, salt and processed oils. However, other Paleo-based diets include "modern" foods which were not available to our cavemen ancestors but support the macronutrient composition of a Paleolithic diet none-the-less. These foods include milk and dairy products, rice, potatoes and some processed oils such as olive oil or canola oil. A Paleo-based diet can be summarized as a diet revolving around the consumption of "real" foods; quality protein and fat in moderation, unlimited vegetables, limited fruits, and the avoidance of all refined carbohydrates and grains containing gluten.

Protein

It's a popular misconception that to build muscle and develop strength, you must eat steak for breakfast, steak for lunch and steak with steak on the side for dinner! This is because meat is popularly believed to be the best source of protein in the diet, and as protein plays an important role in tissue growth and repair, it must therefore be consumed in vast quantities to aid the development of strength. In fact, meat is not necessarily the best source of protein available and excessive amounts of protein from any source do not need to be consumed in order to build muscle. It is resistance training and progressive overload that builds muscle and leads to improvements in strength, not eating extra protein.

Protein is present in your muscles and also in your bones, skin, nails, hair, tendons and arteries. All body proteins are continually being broken down and replaced, and it's through your diet that the protein needed to replenish stores is found. However, not all dietary sources of protein are equal and no natural food is pure protein, unlike the many dietary sources of pure carbohydrate or fat. The quality of the protein you consume is of far greater importance in terms of body building than the quantity, and a mix of different sources is the best way to ensure you gain the optimal quantities of essential amino acids. All proteins are made up of amino acids, some of which can be produced naturally by your body, but others can only be sourced through your diet.

Paleo protein sources include:

Meat

- **Beef** – with the exception of fiber, beef contains most of the nutrients your body needs; calcium, iron, vitamin C, iodine, folate and manganese to name but a few. The vitamin and mineral content of beef depends on the soil grazed. Grass-fed beef provides far greater health benefits than grain-fed beef. Lean beef contains less than five percent fat, half of which is saturated fat.
- **Lamb** – provides a rich source of protein, B vitamins, zinc and iron.
- **Pork** – one of the leanest meat sources of protein; lower in fat than beef and lamb and an excellent source of B vitamins.
- **Offal** – ox liver and calves' liver are rich sources of easily absorbed iron, vitamin A and vitamin B12. Kidneys also provide a rich source of B12 and both liver and kidney are low in fat.
- **Game and Game Birds** – provide excellent sources of protein, with a much lower fat content than domesticated fowl such as chicken. This category includes sources such as venison, rabbit, wild boar and pheasant. They offer a rich source of B vitamins and iron, also potassium and phosphorus. Wild game, when available, represents a chemical free source of protein compared to farmed game, but sources must always be sustainable.

Fish

All forms of fish provide excellent sources of protein however wild varieties offer healthier options than farmed versions. This also applies to **seafood**, with organic sources of crab, oysters, shrimp, scallops, lobster mussels and clams representing healthier choices.

Eggs

Eggs offer an excellent source of protein and healthy fat; a large egg contains around 6-8 grams of protein and 5-7 grams of fat, around 2 grams of which is saturated fat. However, it's recommended that no more than six eggs should be consumed per week due to the high cholesterol content.

Hemp

Provides a good source of protein, a healthy balance of omega-3 and omega-6 essential fatty acids, and contains many B vitamins, vitamin A, calcium, iron, vitamin D, vitamin E, sodium and dietary fiber.

Green leafy vegetables

"Greens" provide a good source of plant protein along with many other health benefits. Good choices include beet greens, collard greens, mustard greens, turnip greens and spinach to name but a few.

Cruciferous vegetables

This group of vegetables includes cabbage, broccoli, kale, cauliflower, rutabaga, kohlrabi and watercress along with others, all of which provide a nutrient-dense source of plant protein.

All of the essential amino acids are present to some degree in most protein foods but to be fully utilized by your body, they must be present in optimal proportions. For example, if you eat a protein food that contains half of the ideal proportions of one of the essential amino acids, your body can only use half of the other essential amino acids present. The other half would be wasted or used by your body as an energy source in the absence of carbohydrates for fuel.

Fats

Good quality fat sources in a Paleo-based diet are the saturated fats provided by grass-fed, organic meat and other organic animal sources including eggs. The preferred cooking fats are tallow, lard, grass-fed butter, ghee, coconut oil, palm oil and perhaps olive oil, although processed oils should be avoided whenever possible and used for dressing foods rather than cooking foods. Some oils contain high levels of omega-6 fatty acids which can cause an inflammatory response in your body. For this reason, most nut and seed oils should be used sparingly. Macadamia nuts offer the lowest levels of omega-6 but alternatives include flax seed oil (linseed oil), walnut oil, avocado oil and canola.

Carbohydrates

Paleo carbohydrate sources are mainly fruits and vegetables. Carbohydrates can be split into two main categories: simple carbohydrates or **sugars**, and complex carbohydrates or **starches**. Starches provide a much slower release of energy compared to sugars, making them the preferred source of fuel for athletes in training. The natural sugar content of most fruits means they must be consumed in moderation to avoid sugar "spikes" and "crashes" whereas the majority of vegetables can be consumed on an "all you can eat" basis.

Good sources of Paleo carbohydrate include:

- **Cassava** – a good source of "starchy" carbohydrate. Also provides calcium, iron, manganese, phosphorus, potassium, B vitamins, vitamin C and dietary fiber. Cassava flour is gluten-free.
- **Taro root** – a starchy vegetable offering a rich source of potassium, and a useful source of calcium, vitamins C and E, B vitamins, manganese, magnesium and copper. Taro leaves are also relatively high in protein.
- **Plantains** – a good low sugar source of starchy carbohydrate, also an excellent source of potassium and dietary fiber, and a useful source of vitamins A and C.
- **Yam** – a good source of vitamin B6, vitamin C, potassium and manganese.
- **White potatoes** – a good source of starchy carbohydrate, protein and fiber. They also provide vitamin C and potassium.
- **Sweet potatoes** – a good source of vitamin B6, vitamin C, vitamin D, iron, magnesium, potassium and beta-carotene.
- **Squash** – a good source of vitamins C and A, and also a useful source of calcium and iron.

In moderation, the following fruits also provide a good source of carbohydrate:

- **Strawberries** - a rich source of vitamin C and also an aid to the absorption of iron from vegetables.

- **Pears** - a good source of vitamin C, potassium, pectin and bioflavonoids. Pectin provides fiber, and bioflavonoids are powerful antioxidants.
- **Mangoes** - a good source of vitamin C and beta-carotene.
- **Bananas** - a rich source of potassium.
- **Apple** – offers a small amount of vitamin C.
- **Peach** – a good source of vitamins A and C.
- **Blueberries** - often described as "the ultimate brain food," blueberries have an antioxidant content of around five times higher than other fruits and vegetables. Research has discovered that a daily serving of 100 grams can stimulate new brain cell growth and slow down the effects of mental ageing.

Both fruits and vegetables provide a healthful source of carbohydrates for energy but the added fiber content of vegetables helps to slow the absorption of sugar and thereby a slower and steadier release of energy is provided. Dark green leafy vegetables are nutritionally dense, making them an ideal source of energy to fuel strength training and muscle building activities.

All carbohydrates are converted by your body into glucose and glycogen before they can be used as fuel. Complex carbohydrates are broken down for use more slowly than simple carbohydrates, meaning they provide a slower release of energy. During weight training exercises, the working muscles are fuelled by glucose in the blood and by glycogen from stores in the liver and in the muscles. Glucose and glycogen are inter-convertible. When your body has a sufficient supply of glucose, carbohydrates are converted to glycogen and stored, but if glucose is in short supply, glycogen is converted to glucose ready for use.

Your body can only store a limited amount of glycogen, so topping up your stores before a training session and replenishing them after a training session is a key factor in maximizing your training efforts. At the end of a training session, your body's ability to store glycogen is elevated. Eating carbohydrate-rich foods in this "glycogen window" of around 30 minutes after exercise is an effective way to replenish your glycogen stores which helps to keep you energized for the rest of the day *and* keeps you powerfully fuelled for the following day's session.

Paleo Smoothies

Smoothies provide the perfect way to increase your useable protein intake, boost your healthy fat intake and top up your glycogen stores, keeping you energized and ready to maximize your performance in every training session. Resistance training creates microscopic damage in your muscles and it's the natural repair and regeneration process that leads to increases in muscle size and strength. A green smoothie made with a combination of fruits and green leafy vegetables can give you a nutritional boost, providing carbohydrates to fuel training and protein to fuel recovery. Adding milk or yogurt from grass-fed sources provides additional protein, with milk containing higher levels of useable protein than meat. The addition of further ingredients such as nuts and seeds can also boost the protein content and provide variety in terms of flavor and texture.

Protein is essentially the body's muscle-builder but adding protein to your diet does not in itself build muscle in body building terms. Resistance training builds muscle, and to train effectively you need to fuel your body with carbohydrates. However, adding protein-rich ingredients to a post-training smoothie can help to promote tissue growth and repair, thereby aiding recovery.

Protein-rich smoothie ingredients include:

Green Leafy Vegetables

- **Beet greens** – the leafy tops of beets contain calcium, iron and beta-carotene, a powerful antioxidant. Calcium is essential for strong bones and teeth, and plays an important role in nerve transmission and muscle functions. Iron is an essential component of hemoglobin, the oxygen carrying pigment in red blood cells, and myoglobin, a similar pigment which stores oxygen in your muscles. Iron is also important in energy metabolism. Antioxidants protect against free radicals, potentially harmful chemicals which are formed by your body as a by-product of its metabolic processes. Related research has found that consuming beets on a regular basis can enhance an athlete's tolerance to high-intensity exercise.
- **Collard greens** – a good source of omega-3 essential fatty acids which have anti-inflammatory properties.
- **Mustard greens** – an excellent source of antioxidant vitamins A, C, E, and vitamin K which plays an essential role in the formation of certain proteins. Also contains carotenes and flavonoids which are powerful antioxidants, and calcium, iron, magnesium, potassium, zinc, selenium and manganese. Magnesium plays an important role in muscle contraction; potassium works with sodium to maintain a fluid and electrolyte balance within the cells and is also essential for the transmission of all nerve impulses; zinc is vital for normal growth and development, and plays an important role in the functioning

of the immune system; selenium is an antioxidant which protects against free radical damage; manganese is a vital component of many enzymes involved in energy production.

- **Turnip greens** – a rich source of beta-carotene, vitamin C, and a useful source of folate, needed for the formation of proteins in the body.
- **Spinach** – a rich source of carotenoids, including antioxidants beta-carotene and lutein. Also contains vitamin C and potassium.

Milk

Organic milk from pasture-fed cows provides two types of protein:

- **Whey protein** – a fast acting protein which helps to reduce the effects of muscle damage immediately after an intense training session.
- **Casein protein** – a slow acting protein which helps to continue the repair process long after the training session.

Both whey and casein proteins are available in powder form, so which is the best smoothie ingredient … powder or milk? Eating a Paleo-based diet is all about eating naturally. Generally, the closer a foodstuff stays to its natural state, the more nutritional value it maintains. For this reason, raw milk is favored over pasteurized milk for those including dairy in a Paleo diet. Milk not only provides a source of high quality protein, but also calcium, zinc and phosphorus. Phosphorus is needed to release energy in cells and plays an essential role in the absorption of many nutrients. **Organic cream** or **organic plain yogurt** can also provide protein, calcium and phosphorus, along with providing a thicker consistency and creamier texture to a smoothie.

Protein powders are convenient to use but the amino acid content, and therefore the useable protein content, varies greatly from product to product so it pays to read labels carefully as powders can be expensive.

Nuts and seeds

- **Flax seeds** - also known as linseeds, provide a good source of protein and are high in omega-3 essential fatty acids. They also contain B vitamins which are involved in the release of energy from food.
- **Pumpkin seeds** – a rich source of protein and fat along with numerous vitamins and minerals including B vitamins, vitamin E, copper, manganese, potassium, calcium, magnesium, iron, zinc and selenium. Copper is present in many enzymes which protect against free radicals and helps the body to absorb iron from food.
- **Sunflower seeds** – provide protein along with vitamin E, selenium, magnesium and copper.
- **Almonds** – provide protein along with calcium, magnesium, potassium, vitamin E and other antioxidants.
- **Cashews** – a good source of protein and rich in iron, phosphorus, selenium, zinc and magnesium.
- **Walnuts** – provide protein and also a rich source of omega-3 fatty acids.

The Benefits of Smoothies for Strength Training

Building muscle and developing strength and power is all about progressively overloading your muscles to promote adaptation. Using an appropriate training plan, the more your body is asked to do, the more it becomes able to do; your body adapts to the repeated demands being placed upon it.

A carbohydrate-rich smoothie can provide a pre-training boost to your glycogen stores and a glycogen replenishing "recovery" boost after an intense training session. Any combination of fruits in a smoothie will provide energy-giving carbohydrates so your choice is a matter of personal taste. The antioxidant properties of many fruits can also help to reduce the effects of muscular damage generated through training. As a general guide, fruits with orange or dark yellow flesh provide a good source of beta-carotene, and fruits with red flesh offer a good source of lycopene. The combination of beta-carotene and lycopene is thought to be very effective in terms of protecting your body against free radicals.

Combining fruits and vegetables in a green smoothie provides an even greater nutritional boost and the added fiber content helps to give a slower release of energy. Ideal post-training smoothie ingredients to boost recovery and replenish glycogen stores might include:

- **Green leafy vegetables of your choice** - leafy vegetables provide carbohydrates and protein to promote muscle growth and repair.
- **Fruits of your choice** - fresh or frozen fruits provide carbohydrates to replenish your glycogen stores, antioxidants to give your immune system a boost, and sweetness to please your taste buds.
- **Organic raw milk, cream or plain Greek yogurt** - provides whey protein to reduce the effects of muscle damage and promote repair after an intense training session.
- **Flax seeds, coconut oil, or almond butter** (organic, grass-fed source) - these provide an additional source of fat and add flavor and texture.

Adding fresh herbs to a green smoothie can also add a flavorsome twist along with providing further nutritional benefits. Popular choices include:

- **Parsley** - one cup of parsley contains 2 grams of protein. It is also rich in calcium and provides iron, copper, magnesium, potassium, zinc, phosphorus, beta-carotene and vitamin C.
- **Dill** – adds a sweet flavor to a smoothie and contains calcium, iron, manganese, vitamin C, and beta-carotene.

- **Sorrel** - provides iron, magnesium and calcium.
- **Basil** - provides beta-carotene, iron, potassium, copper, manganese and magnesium
- **Coriander** - provides a mild, peppery flavor along with anti-inflammatory properties, vitamin C, iron and magnesium.

Some flavorsome green smoothie combinations that may help to maximize your training efforts include:

Spinach with strawberries - the sweetness of the fruit overrides the flavor of the spinach, providing an antioxidant-rich smoothie.

Kale with oranges - kale contains iron, calcium, vitamin C and beta-carotene, with citrus fruits also providing a rich source of vitamin C and antioxidants.

Collard greens with apple and dates - collard greens contain omega-3 fatty acids, thereby providing anti-inflammatory properties, and dates are good source of iron and calcium.

Tried and tested smoothie recipes are a great way to get started but there are virtually no limits to the flavorsome and nutritious combinations that can be created. Creating Paleo-based smoothies is simple – if it's fresh (or frozen at source), organic, high quality and natural, it's a good choice. If it's in a box, it's not a good choice! Paleo foods are *real* foods, so make your smoothies with foods you chop, slice, prepare and blend from scratch. The energizing nutritional benefits are well worth the effort.

General Information about Your Smoothies

These smoothies are divided into 2 categories, each designed to meet the nutritional needs of cyclist in two moments:

Pre-training smoothies;

Post-training smoothies.

The great majority of the ingredients in these recipes has a low Glycemic Index.

When the recipes call for fruit juice, always choose one that is made of pure fruit.

If you can't find the fresh fruit you need for a recipe, feel free to replace it with frozen. Frozen fruits have the same nutritional content as the corresponding fresh fruits.

You can adjust the consistency of your smoothie adding some ice cubes to the recipe before blending and/or straining before serving.

Pre-Training Smoothies

These smoothies were developed to provide an adequate amount of Carbohydrates for a 150 pounds person. You can adjust the amount of carbohydrates by adding, for each extra 5 pounds of body weight, one of the following:

½ tsp. of. of raw honey;

1 tbsp. of. of flax seeds;

1 tsp. of. of seeded raisins;

½ tbsp. of. of dried apricots;

3 ½ tbsp. of grass-fed milk;

2 ½ tbsp. of organic yogurt.

1. Pineapple and Pitaya Smoothie

Preparation time	5 minutes
Ready time	5 minutes
Serves	1
Serving quantity/unit	530 G / 19 Ounces
Calories	300 Cal
Total Fat	1g
Cholesterol	3 mg
Sodium	50 mg
Total Carbohydrates	68 g
Dietary fibers	3g
Sugars	58 g
Protein	7g

Prepare your smoothie combining the following ingredients in a food processor:

- 1 ½ cups of pineapple
- 1 cup of pure pitaya juice
- ¼ cup of organic Greek yogurt
- 1 tsp. of raw honey

2. Banana, Tangerine and Carrot Smoothie

Preparation time	5 minutes
Ready time	5 minutes
Serves	1
Serving quantity/unit	430 G / 15 Ounces
Calories	316 Cal
Total Fat	5 g
Cholesterol	11 mg
Sodium	100 mg
Total Carbohydrates	72 g
Dietary fibers	10g
Sugars	46 g
Protein	4g

Prepare your smoothie combining the following ingredients in a food processor:

- 1 cup of carrot
- ¾ cup of tangerines, (mandarin oranges)
- 1 cup of banana
- ¼ cup of organic cream
- 1 tsp. of honey

3. Currant and Apricot Smoothie

Preparation time	5 minutes
Ready time	5 minutes
Serves	1
Serving quantity/unit	436 G / 15 Ounces
Calories	319 Cal
Total Fat	3g
Cholesterol	10 mg
Sodium	53 mg
Total Carbohydrates	68 g
Dietary fibers	11 g
Sugars	58 g
Protein	10g

Prepare your smoothie combining the following ingredients in a food processor:

- 1 cup of currants
- 1 cup of apricots
- ¼ cup of dried apricots
- 1 tsp. of honey
- ½ cup of grass-fed milk

4. Orange and Blueberries Smoothie

Preparation time	5 minutes
Ready time	5 minutes
Serves	1
Serving quantity/unit	470 G / 17 Ounces
Calories	287 Cal
Total Fat	2 g
Cholesterol	0 mg
Sodium	76 mg
Total Carbohydrates	69 g
Dietary fibers	5 g
Sugars	54 g
Protein	3g

Prepare your smoothie combining the following ingredients in a food processor:

- 1 cup of blueberries
- ¾ cup of orange juice
- ½ cup of almond milk
- 1 ½ tsps. of honey
- 2 tbsps. of raisins

5. Melon and Blackberries Smoothie

Preparation time	5 minutes
Ready time	5 minutes
Serves	1
Serving quantity/unit	510 G / 18 Ounces
Calories	313 Cal
Total Fat	5 g
Cholesterol	11 mg
Sodium	60 mg
Total Carbohydrates	69 g
Dietary fibers	17g
Sugars	46 g
Protein	6 g

Prepare your smoothie combining the following ingredients in a food processor:

- 1 ½ cups of melon
- 1 ½ cups of blackberries
- ¼ cup of prunes
- ¼ cup of organic cream

6. Peach and Papaya Smoothie

Preparation time	5 minutes
Ready time	5 minutes
Serves	1
Serving quantity/unit	520 G /18 Ounces
Calories	300 Cal
Total Fat	2 g
Cholesterol	3 mg
Sodium	26 mg
Total Carbohydrates	68 g
Dietary fibers	8 g
Sugars	50 g
Protein	9 g

Prepare your smoothie combining the following ingredients in a food processor:

- 1 cup of peach
- 1 ½ cups of papaya
- ½ cup of banana
- 2 tsps. of honey
- ¼ cup of organic Greek yogurt

7. Strawberry and Currant Smoothie with Beet

Preparation time	5 minutes
Ready time	5 minutes
Serves	1
Serving quantity/unit	480 G / 17 Ounces
Calories	299 Cal
Total Fat	3 g
Cholesterol	10 mg
Sodium	52 mg
Total Carbohydrates	69 g
Dietary fibers	7g
Sugars	53 g
Protein	6g

Prepare your smoothie combining the following ingredients in a food processor:

- 1 ¼ cups of pear
- 1 pomegranate, around 150g/5oz.
- ½ cup of organic raw grass-fed milk
- 1 tsp. of honey

8. Coconut and Loquat Smoothie

Preparation time	5 minutes
Ready time	5 minutes
Serves	1
Serving quantity/unit	510 G / 18 Ounces
Calories	497 Cal
Total Fat	28 g
Cholesterol	0 mg
Sodium	22 mg
Total Carbohydrates	68 g
Dietary fibers	9g
Sugars	28 g
Protein	4 g

Prepare your smoothie combining the following ingredients in a food processor:

- 2 cups of loquat
- ½ cup of mango
- ½ cup of coconut milk
- 2 tsps. of honey

9. Grape and Watermelon Smoothie

Preparation time	5 minutes
Ready time	5 minutes
Serves	1
Serving quantity/unit	415 G / 14 Ounces
Calories	313 Cal
Total Fat	3 g
Cholesterol	10 mg
Sodium	59 mg
Total Carbohydrates	71 g
Dietary fibers	3 g
Sugars	59 g
Protein	7g

Prepare your smoothie combining the following ingredients in a food processor:

- 1 cup of grape
- 1 cup of watermelon
- 1/3 cup of raisins
- ½ cup of grass-fed milk

10. Strawberry and Pear Smoothie

Preparation time	5 minutes
Ready time	5 minutes
Serves	1
Serving quantity/unit	470 G / 17 Ounces
Calories	320 Cal
Total Fat	7 g
Cholesterol	23 mg
Sodium	44 mg
Total Carbohydrates	68 g
Dietary fibers	12g
Sugars	45 g
Protein	3 g

Prepare your smoothie combining the following ingredients in a food processor:

- ¾ cup of strawberries
- 2 cups of pear
- ½ cup of organic cream
- 1 tsp. of honey

11. Coconut and Lemon Smoothie with Watercress

Preparation time	5 minutes
Ready time	5 minutes
Serves	1
Serving quantity/unit	420 G / 15 Ounces
Calories	443 Cal
Total Fat	16 g
Cholesterol	6 mg
Sodium	62 mg
Total Carbohydrates	68 g
Dietary fibers	8g
Sugars	44 g
Protein	15g

Prepare your smoothie combining the following ingredients in a food processor:

- ½ cup of coconut
- ¼ cup of lemon juice
- 1 cup of banana
- 1 cup of watercress
- 1 tbsp. of honey
- ½ cup of organic Greek yogurt

12. Passion fruit and Apricot Smoothie with Broccoli

Preparation time	5 minutes
Ready time	5 minutes
Serves	1
Serving quantity/unit	520 G / 19 Ounces
Calories	308 Cal
Total Fat	3 g
Cholesterol	0 mg
Sodium	153 mg
Total Carbohydrates	70 g
Dietary fibers	24g
Sugars	40 g
Protein	8g

Prepare your smoothie combining the following ingredients in a food processor:

- ¾ cup of passion fruit
- 1 cup of apricot
- ½ cup of broccoli
- ½ cup of almond milk

13. Plum and Strawberry Smoothie

Preparation time	5 minutes
Ready time	5 minutes
Serves	1
Serving quantity/unit	400 G / 14 Ounces
Calories	297 Cal
Total Fat	4 g
Cholesterol	11 mg
Sodium	22 mg
Total Carbohydrates	68 g
Dietary fibers	9 g
Sugars	46 g
Protein	4g

Prepare your smoothie combining the following ingredients in a food processor:

- 1 cup of plums
- 1/3 cup of prunes
- 1 cup of strawberries
- ¼ cup of organic cream

14. Cherry, Beetroot and Lemon Smoothie

Preparation time	5 minutes
Ready time	5 minutes
Serves	1
Serving quantity/unit	570 G / 20 Ounces
Calories	313
Total Fat	3 g
Cholesterol	3 mg
Sodium	150 mg
Total Carbohydrates	69 g
Dietary fibers	10 g
Sugars	55 g
Protein	13g

Prepare your smoothie combining the following ingredients in a food processor:

- 1 cup of beet
- 2 cups of cherries
- ¼ cup of lemon juice
- ¼ cup of organic Greek yogurt

15. Kiwi and Guava Smoothie with Cabbage

Preparation time	5 minutes
Ready time	5 minutes
Serves	1
Serving quantity/unit	580 G / 20 Ounces
Calories	346 Cal
Total Fat	6 g
Cholesterol	10 mg
Sodium	67 mg
Total Carbohydrates	69 g
Dietary fibers	20g
Sugars	45 g
Protein	13g

Prepare your smoothie combining the following ingredients in a food processor:

- 1 ½ cups of guava
- 1 cup of kiwi
- ½ cup of cabbage
- ½ cup of grass-fed milk

16. Apple and Raspberry Smoothie

Preparation time	5 minutes
Ready time	5 minutes
Serves	1
Serving quantity/unit	500 G / 18 Ounces
Calories	427 Cal
Total Fat	17 g
Cholesterol	0 mg
Sodium	74 mg
Total Carbohydrates	69 g
Dietary fibers	17g
Sugars	46 g
Protein	9 g

Prepare your smoothie combining the following ingredients in a food processor:

- 2 cups of apple
- 1 cup of raspberries
- ½ cup of almond milk
- 5 tbsps. of almonds
- 2 tsps. of honey

17. Watermelon and Banana Smoothie

Preparation time	5 minutes
Ready time	5 minutes
Serves	1
Serving quantity/unit	530 G / 19 Ounces
Calories	342 Cal
Total Fat	3 g
Cholesterol	6 mg
Sodium	41 mg
Total Carbohydrates	70 g
Dietary fibers	7g
Sugars	44 g
Protein	15 g

Prepare your smoothie combining the following ingredients in a food processor:

- 1 ¼ cups of watermelon
- 1 ½ cups of banana
- ½ cup of organic Greek yogurt

18. Pineapple and Pear Smoothie

Preparation time	5 minutes
Ready time	5 minutes
Serves	1
Serving quantity/unit	520 G / 19 Ounces
Calories	290 Cal
Total Fat	4 g
Cholesterol	11 mg
Sodium	26 mg
Total Carbohydrates	69 g
Dietary fibers	11g
Sugars	47 g
Protein	2g

Prepare your smoothie combining the following ingredients in a food processor:

- 1 cup of pineapple
- 1 ¾ cups of pear
- ¼ cup of organic cream
- ½ tsp. of honey
- 3 ice cubes

Post-Training Smoothies

These smoothies were created with great combinations of carbohydrates and protein sources which will be essential to give your body the right nutrients, enhancing its recovery after your workout. Also in these recipes, if you weight more than 150 pounds, it is better to adjust the nutritional content of your smoothie by adding, for each extra 5 pounds of body weight, one of these:

1 tbsp. of. of almonds;

1 tbsp. of. of nuts mixture;

1 tbsp. of. of flaxseeds;

1tbsp. of. of sesame seeds;

2 tbsp. of grass-fed milk;

2 tbsp. of organic yogurt.

19. Kiwi and Blackberry Smoothie

Preparation time	5 minutes
Ready time	5 minutes
Serves	1
Serving quantity/unit	560 G / 19 Ounces
Calories	488 Cal
Total Fat	16 g
Cholesterol	6 mg
Sodium	47 mg
Total Carbohydrates	74 g
Dietary fibers	19 g
Sugars	48 g
Protein	21 g

Prepare your smoothie combining the following ingredients in a food processor:

- 1 ½ cups of kiwi
- 1 cup of blackberries
- ½ cup of organic Greek yogurt
- ¼ cup of almonds
- 2 tsps. of honey

20. Cherry and Tangerine Smoothie

Preparation time	5 minutes
Ready time	5 minutes
Serves	1
Serving quantity/unit	580 G / 20 Ounces
Calories	374 Cal
Total Fat	4 g
Cholesterol	9 mg
Sodium	65 mg
Total Carbohydrates	69 g
Dietary fibers	6g
Sugars	63 g
Protein	21g

Prepare your smoothie combining the following ingredients in a food processor:

- 1 ½ cups of Cherries
- ¾ cup of tangerines
- ¾ cup of organic Greek yogurt
- 2 tsps. of honey

21. Watermelon Smoothie with Romaine Lettuce and Almonds

Preparation time	5 minutes
Ready time	5 minutes
Serves	1
Serving quantity/unit	530 G / 19 Ounces
Calories	494 Cal
Total Fat	17 g
Cholesterol	6 mg
Sodium	51 mg
Total Carbohydrates	68 g
Dietary fibers	16g
Sugars	43 g
Protein	21g

Prepare your smoothie combining the following ingredients in a food processor:

- 2 cups of watermelon
- 1 cup of romaine lettuce
- ¼ cup of dried cherries
- 5 tbsps. of almonds
- ½ cup of organic Greek yogurt

22. Melon and Fig Smoothie

Preparation time	5 minutes
Ready time	5 minutes
Serves	1
Serving quantity/unit	540 G / 19 Ounces
Calories	367 Cal
Total Fat	5 g
Cholesterol	11 mg
Sodium	117 mg
Total Carbohydrates	70 g
Dietary fibers	8g
Sugars	62 g
Protein	18g

Prepare your smoothie combining the following ingredients in a food processor:

- 2 cups of melon
- ¼ cup of fig
- ½ cup of organic Greek yogurt
- ¼ cup of grass-fed milk
- 1 tsp. of honey

23. Cherry Smoothie with Kale and Flax Seeds

Preparation time	5 minutes
Ready time	5 minutes
Serves	1
Serving quantity/unit	600 G / 21 Ounces
Calories	390 Cal
Total Fat	10 g
Cholesterol	20 mg
Sodium	145 mg
Total Carbohydrates	68 g
Dietary fibers	10g
Sugars	51 g
Protein	17g

Prepare your smoothie combining the following ingredients in a food processor:

- 2 cups of cherries
- 1 ½ cups of kale
- 1 cup of organic grass-fed milk
- 1 tbsp. of flax seed

24. Peach Smoothie with Beet Greens

Preparation time	5 minutes
Ready time	5 minutes
Serves	1
Serving quantity/unit	510 G / 18 Ounces
Calories	437 Cal
Total Fat	13 g
Cholesterol	6 mg
Sodium	209 mg
Total Carbohydrates	70 g
Dietary fibers	11g
Sugars	61 g
Protein	19g

Prepare your smoothie combining the following ingredients in a food processor:

- 1 ½ cups of peach
- ¼ cup of dried apricots
- 2 cups of beet greens
- ½ cup of organic Greek yogurt
- 2 tbsps. of pecans
- 2 tsps. of honey

25. Raspberry and Prunes Smoothie

Preparation time	5 minutes
Ready time	5 minutes
Serves	1
Serving quantity/unit	480 G / 17 Ounces
Calories	378 Cal
Total Fat	6 g
Cholesterol	15 mg
Sodium	90 mg
Total Carbohydrates	69 g
Dietary fibers	16g
Sugars	41 g
Protein	19g

Prepare your smoothie combining the following ingredients in a food processor:

- 1 ½ cups of raspberries
- 1/3 cup of prunes
- ½ cup of grass-fed milk
- ½ cup of organic Greek yogurt

26. Guava and Cucumber Smoothie

Preparation time	5 minutes
Ready time	5 minutes
Serves	1
Serving quantity/unit	600 G / 21 Ounces
Calories	458 Cal
Total Fat	16 g
Cholesterol	15 mg
Sodium	83 mg
Total Carbohydrates	70 g
Dietary fibers	20 g
Sugars	49 g
Protein	19 g

Prepare your smoothie combining the following ingredients in a food processor:

- 2 cups of guava
- ½ cup of cucumber
- ¾ cup of organic grass-fed milk
- 3 tbsps. of almonds
- 1 ½ tsps. of honey

27. Apricot and Lemon Smoothie

Preparation time	5 minutes
Ready time	5 minutes
Serves	1
Serving quantity/unit	630 G / 22 Ounces
Calories	557 Cal
Total Fat	27.4 g
Cholesterol	10 mg
Sodium	55 mg
Total Carbohydrates	70 g
Dietary fibers	14 g
Sugars	51 g
Protein	20 g

Prepare your smoothie combining the following ingredients in a food processor:

- ½ cup of dried apricots
- 2 cups of apricot
- ¼ cup of lemon juice
- ½ cup of grass-fed milk
- ½ cup of almonds
- 1 tsp. of honey

28. Passion fruit and Coconut Smoothie

Preparation time	5 minutes
Ready time	5 minutes
Serves	1
Serving quantity/unit	410 G / 14 Ounces
Calories	456 Cal
Total Fat	17 g
Cholesterol	6 mg
Sodium	111 mg
Total Carbohydrates	66 g
Dietary fibers	28 g
Sugars	34 g
Protein	18 g

Prepare your smoothie combining the following ingredients in a food processor:

- ½ cup of coconut
- 1 cup of passion fruit pulp
- ½ cup of Greek yogurt
- 3 ice cubes

29. Apple and Loquat Smoothie with Nuts

Preparation time	5 minutes
Ready time	5 minutes
Serves	1
Serving quantity/unit	550 G / 19 Ounces
Calories	550 Cal
Total Fat	27 g
Cholesterol	20 mg
Sodium	109 mg
Total Carbohydrates	69 g
Dietary fibers	8 g
Sugars	43 g
Protein	17g

Prepare your smoothie combining the following ingredients in a food processor:

- 1 ½ cups of apple
- ½ cup of loquats
- ¼ cup of cashews
- 1 cup of grass-fed milk
- 2 tbsps. of almonds
- 2 tsps. of honey

30. Papaya and Grape Smoothie

Preparation time	5 minutes
Ready time	5 minutes
Serves	1
Serving quantity/unit	560 G /20 Ounces
Calories	366 Cal
Total Fat	4 g
Cholesterol	9 mg
Sodium	68 mg
Total Carbohydrates	68 g
Dietary fibers	7 g
Sugars	52 g
Protein	20g

Prepare your smoothie combining the following ingredients in a food processor:

- 2 cups of papaya
- 1 cup of grapes
- 2 ½ tbsps. of raisins
- ¾ cup of organic Greek yogurt

31. Blueberry Smoothie

Preparation time	5 minutes
Ready time	5 minutes
Serves	1
Serving quantity/unit	590 G / 21 Ounces
Calories	582 Cal
Total Fat	29 g
Cholesterol	20 mg
Sodium	104 mg
Total Carbohydrates	70 g
Dietary fibers	13 g
Sugars	49 g
Protein	20 g

Prepare your smoothie combining the following ingredients in a food processor:

- 2 cups of blueberries
- 1 cup of grass-fed milk
- ½ cup of almonds
- 1 tsp. of honey

32. Watermelon and Mango Smoothie

Preparation time	5 minutes
Ready time	5 minutes
Serves	1
Serving quantity/unit	600 G / 21 Ounces
Calories	372 Cal
Total Fat	4 g
Cholesterol	9 mg
Sodium	63 mg
Total Carbohydrates	70 g
Dietary fibers	6g
Sugars	62 g
Protein	19g

Prepare your smoothie combining the following ingredients in a food processor:

- 1 ¾ cups of mango
- 1 cup of watermelon
- ¾ cup of Greek yogurt
- ½ tsp. of honey

33. Pitaya and Pear Juice with Flax Seeds and Almonds

Preparation time	5 minutes
Ready time	5 minutes
Serves	1
Serving quantity/unit	540 G / 19 Ounces
Calories	456 Cal
Total Fat	15 g
Cholesterol	8 mg
Sodium	61 mg
Total Carbohydrates	69 g
Dietary fibers	13 g
Sugars	47 g
Protein	18g

Prepare your smoothie combining the following ingredients in a food processor:

- ½ cup of pure pitaya juice
- 1 ¾ cups of pear
- 1 tbsp. of flax seed
- 3 tbsps. of almonds
- 1 tbsp. of organic cream
- ½ cup of organic Greek yogurt

34. Mango and Pineapple Smoothie with Spinach

Preparation time	5 minutes
Ready time	5 minutes
Serves	1
Serving quantity/unit	600 G / 21 Ounces
Calories	427 Cal
Total Fat	10 g
Cholesterol	6 mg
Sodium	92 mg
Total Carbohydrates	75 g
Dietary fibers	9g
Sugars	59 g
Protein	18g

Prepare your smoothie combining the following ingredients in a food processor:

- 1 ½ cups of pineapple
- 1 cup of mango
- 2 cups of spinach
- ½ cup of organic Greek yogurt
- 1 tbsp. of cashews
- 1 tbsp. of almonds
- 1 tsp. of honey

35. Pear and Apple Smoothie With Collard Greens

Preparation time	5 minutes
Ready time	5 minutes
Serves	1
Serving quantity/unit	660 G / 23 Ounces
Calories	377 Cal
Total Fat	6 g
Cholesterol	18 mg
Sodium	104 mg
Total Carbohydrates	79 g
Dietary fibers	12g
Sugars	53 g
Protein	11g

Prepare your smoothie combining the following ingredients in a food processor:

- 1 cup of pear
- 1 cup of apple
- ¾ cup of banana
- 1 cup of collard greens
- 1 cup of grass-fed milk

36. Fennel, Kiwi and Banana Smoothie

Preparation time	5 minutes
Ready time	5 minutes
Serves	1
Serving quantity/unit	670 G / 24 Ounces
Calories	627 Cal
Total Fat	37 g
Cholesterol	15 mg
Sodium	105 mg
Total Carbohydrates	69 g
Dietary fibers	17g
Sugars	41 g
Protein	18g

Prepare your smoothie combining the following ingredients in a food processor:

- 1 cup of kiwi
- ¼ cup of banana
- 1 ¼ cups of strawberries
- ½ cup of fennel
- ¾ cup of organic grass-fed milk
- 4 tbsps. of almonds
- 4 tbsps. of pecans

Exclusive Bonus Download: 100 Bodybuilding Tips

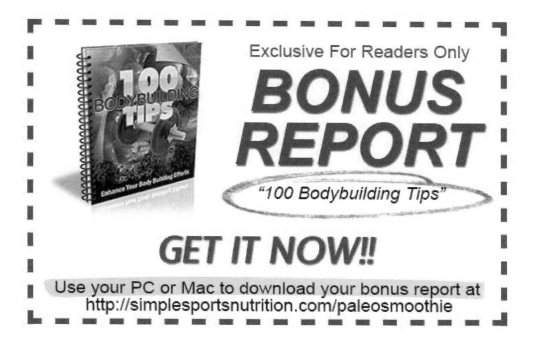

Download your bonus, please visit the download link above from your PC or MAC. To open PDF files, visit http://get.adobe.com/reader/ to download the reader if it's not already installed on your PC or Mac. To open ZIP files, you may need to download WinZip from http://www.winzip.com. This download is for PC or Mac ONLY and might not be downloadable to kindle.

People all over the world, not just men, are interested in bulking up through bodybuilding exercises. This area used to be the exclusive domain of men, but now women are becoming serious bodybuilders, whether competing in body sculpting competitions or getting more muscles to lift more weight. Whatever the reason, bodybuilding is one of the hot topics being researched online today.

But just like any exercise or diet routine, bodybuilding requires discipline. You need to take stock of yourself first to see if you have the commitment that it's going to take. " 100 Bodybuilding Tips " will show you how to attain the right mindset, how to prepare yourself physically, ways to burn fat and build cardio strength, and pitfalls to avoid in establishing a bodybuilding routine. These tips contain the information that you'll need to get started on a serious regimen, all the while avoiding injury and developing muscle mass safely in harmony with your body's processes. You'll get information about which exercises produce which results, and how to avoid the common myths that many people believe about gaining muscle through bodybuilding.

People begin to lose muscle mass as they approach middle age. Many people who enjoyed the benefits of strength in their youth find themselves with backaches and other ailments which could be alleviated with stronger, healthier muscles. Whether you want to be on the cover of a fitness magazine or just enjoy a higher quality of life, get " 100 Bodybuilding Tips " and learn how to make a change in your life today.

Visit the URL above to download this guide and start achieving your weight loss and fitness goals NOW

One Last Thing...

Thank you so much for reading my book. I hope you really liked it. As you probably know, many people look at the reviews on Amazon before they decide to purchase a book. If you liked the book, could you please take a minute to leave a review with your feedback? 60 seconds is all I'm asking for, and it would mean the world to me.

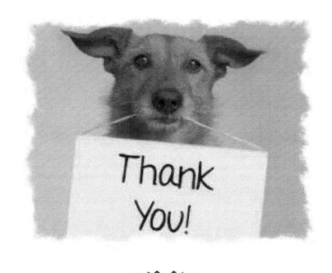

Books by Lars Andersen

The Smoothies for Runners Book

Juices for Runners

Smoothies for Cyclists

Juices for Cyclists

Palio Diet for Cyclists

Smoothies for Triathletes

Juices for Triathletes

Palio Diet for Triathletes

Smoothies for Strength

<u>Juices for Strength</u>

<u>Palio Diet for Strength</u>

<u>Palio Diet Smoothies for Strength</u>

<u>Smoothies for Golfers</u>

<u>Juices for Golfers</u>

About the Author

Lars Andersen is a sports author, nutritional researcher and fitness enthusiast. In his spare time he participates in competitive running, swimming and cycling events and enjoys hiking with his two border collies.

Lars Andersen

Published by Nordic Standard Publishing

Atlanta, Georgia USA

NORDICSTANDARD
PUBLISHING

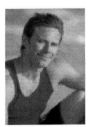